HEAVY METAL
DETOX
COOKBOOK

Dr. Kimberly Carlos

2 |

TABLE OF CONTENT

INTRODUCTION

Sarah had always been an adventurous spirit, embracing life with vigor and excitement. But as the years passed, she began to feel sluggish, her energy waning, and her health deteriorating. After consulting with several doctors, she decided to take matters into her own hands and explore alternative approaches to rejuvenate her body.

One day, while researching holistic health remedies, Sarah stumbled upon the concept of heavy metal detox diets. Intrigued, she delved deeper into the subject and learned about the potential dangers of heavy metal accumulation in the body from sources like contaminated water, fish, and dental fillings.

Determined to reclaim her vitality, Sarah embarked on a journey to detoxify her body. She revamped her diet, incorporating a wide array of foods known for their detoxifying properties, such as leafy greens, garlic, cilantro, and chlorella. She also eliminated processed foods and sugary snacks from her daily routine.

As weeks turned into months, Sarah began to notice a remarkable transformation. Her energy levels soared, and she felt more mentally alert than ever before. Her skin, once dull and tired-looking, now had a healthy glow. Sarah's friends and family couldn't believe the change in her. They commented on her newfound radiance and vitality.

Sarah's dedication to her heavy metal detox diet didn't just improve her physical health; it also boosted her mental well-being. She felt lighter, both physically and emotionally, as if a burden had been lifted from her shoulders. Her newfound clarity of mind allowed her to pursue her passions and dreams with renewed vigor.

Sarah's inspiring journey not only transformed her life but also served as a testament to the power of holistic health approaches. Through her experience, she learned that taking charge of one's health could lead to a vibrant and fulfilling life. She had discovered the incredible potential of a heavy metal detox diet, proving that sometimes, the path to well-being lies in unconventional choices and a commitment to self-care.

CHAPTER ONE

Following a Heavy Metal Detox Diet with Benefits

Following a heavy metal detox diet can offer various benefits by helping your body eliminate harmful heavy metals and promoting overall health. Here's a step-by-step guide on how to follow such a diet effectively:

1. Consult a healthcare professional: Before starting any detox diet, consult with a healthcare professional or a registered dietitian to ensure it's appropriate for your individual health needs and goals. They can help you tailor the diet to your specific circumstances.

2. Identify sources of heavy metal exposure: Determine potential sources of heavy metal exposure in your life, such as contaminated water, fish high in mercury, dental fillings, or exposure to industrial pollutants. Reducing exposure to these sources is a crucial part of the detoxification process.

3. Choose detoxifying foods: Incorporate foods known for their heavy metal detoxifying properties into your diet. Some of these include:

- Leafy greens: Spinach, kale, and cilantro can help bind to heavy metals and aid in their elimination.
- Cruciferous vegetables: Broccoli, cauliflower, and cabbage support liver function, which is essential for detoxification.
- Garlic and onions: These sulfur-rich foods enhance the body's detoxification pathways.
- Chlorella and spirulina: These algae are believed to help bind to heavy metals and facilitate their removal.
- Turmeric and ginger: These spices have anti-inflammatory and detoxifying properties.

4. Prioritize clean, organic foods: Choose organic produce and high-quality, clean sources of protein, such as grass-fed meat and wild-caught fish, to reduce your exposure to pesticides and contaminants.

5. Hydrate with clean water: Drink filtered or purified water to avoid heavy metal contamination from tap water. Consider investing in a quality water filter.

6. Eliminate processed and sugary foods: Cut out processed foods, sugary snacks, and drinks from your diet, as they can contribute to inflammation and hinder the detoxification process.

7. Be mindful of seafood choices: When consuming fish, opt for low-mercury options like salmon, sardines, and trout. Avoid fish high in mercury, such as swordfish, shark, and king mackerel.

8. Support your liver: Your liver plays a central role in detoxification. To support it, limit alcohol intake and avoid overloading it with toxins like excessive caffeine and medications.

9. Stay consistent: Consistency is key to achieving the benefits of a heavy metal detox diet. Make these dietary changes part of your daily routine and maintain them over time.

10. Consider supplements: Some individuals may benefit from supplements like N-acetylcysteine (NAC) or alpha-lipoic acid, which can support detoxification pathways. However, consult with a healthcare professional before taking any supplements.

11. Monitor your progress: Regularly assess your health and energy levels to gauge the effectiveness of the detox diet. Make adjustments as needed in consultation with your healthcare provider.

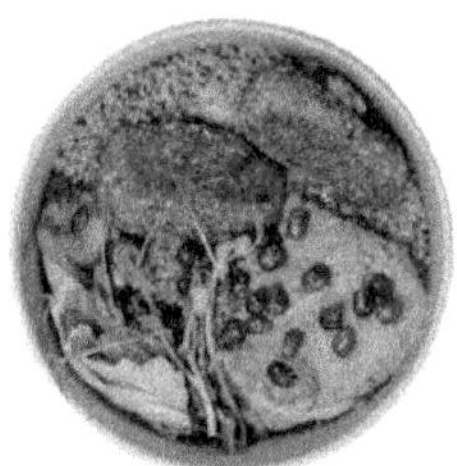 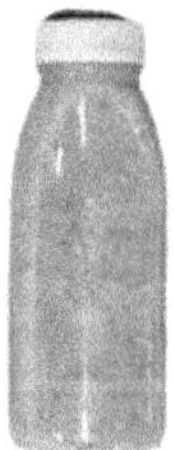

CHAPTER TWO

14-Day Heavy Metal Detox Meal Plan

Day 1

- Breakfast: Green smoothie with spinach, kale, banana, and spirulina.
- Lunch: Grilled chicken salad with mixed greens, cherry tomatoes, and a lemon-tahini dressing.
- Dinner: Baked salmon with steamed broccoli and quinoa.
- Snack: Carrot and cucumber sticks with hummus.

Day 2

- Breakfast: Oatmeal topped with blueberries, chia seeds, and a drizzle of honey.
- Lunch: Lentil and vegetable soup with a side of mixed greens.
- Dinner: Stir-fried tofu with broccoli, bell peppers, and a ginger-garlic sauce served over brown rice.
- Snack: Greek yogurt with sliced strawberries.

Day 3

- Breakfast: Scrambled eggs with spinach and a side of avocado.
- Lunch: Chickpea salad with diced cucumber, red onion, and a lemon-turmeric dressing.
- Dinner: Baked cod with roasted Brussels sprouts and quinoa.
- Snack: Mixed nuts and dried cranberries.

Day 4

- Breakfast: Smoothie bowl with acai, banana, almond milk, and topped with granola, sliced kiwi, and coconut flakes.
- Lunch: Quinoa and black bean bowl with diced tomatoes, corn, and cilantro-lime dressing.
- Dinner: Grilled shrimp with steamed asparagus and mashed sweet potatoes.
- Snack: Sliced apples with almond butter.

Day 5

- Breakfast: Chia seed pudding with raspberries and a sprinkle of flaxseeds.
- Lunch: Spinach and kale salad with grilled chicken, strawberries, and a balsamic vinaigrette.
- Dinner: Baked trout with sautéed spinach and quinoa.
- Snack: Celery sticks with peanut butter.

Day 6

- Breakfast: Greek yogurt parfait with layers of berries and honey.
- Lunch: Lentil and vegetable stir-fry with a sesame-soy sauce served over brown rice.
- Dinner: Baked chicken breast with roasted sweet potatoes and green beans.
- Snack: Trail mix with almonds, walnuts, and dark chocolate chips.

Day 7

- Breakfast: Whole-grain toast with smashed avocado and a poached egg.
- Lunch: Chickpea and quinoa salad with diced cucumber, red pepper, and a lemon-tahini dressing.

- Dinner: Baked halibut with steamed broccoli and couscous.
- Snack: Sliced cucumbers with tzatziki dip.

Day 8

- Breakfast: Green smoothie with kale, banana, almond milk, and a scoop of chlorella powder.
- Lunch: Quinoa and black bean salad with diced red onion, corn, and a lime-cilantro dressing.
- Dinner: Grilled salmon with asparagus and a side of brown rice.
- Snack: Sliced bell peppers with guacamole.

Day 9

- Breakfast: Overnight oats made with rolled oats, almond milk, grated apple, and a sprinkle of cinnamon.
- Lunch: Mixed greens salad with grilled tofu, cherry tomatoes, and a balsamic vinaigrette.
- Dinner: Baked cod with roasted Brussels sprouts and quinoa.
- Snack: Mixed nuts and dried apricots.

Day 10

- Breakfast: Greek yogurt parfait with layers of pineapple chunks and honey.
- Lunch: Lentil soup with a side of steamed broccoli.
- Dinner: Baked chicken breast with sautéed spinach and mashed sweet potatoes.
- Snack: Sliced pear with almond butter.

Day 11

- Breakfast: Smoothie bowl with a blend of mixed berries, almond milk, and topped with granola, sliced banana, and chia seeds.
- Lunch: Chickpea and vegetable stir-fry with a ginger-soy sauce served over brown rice.
- Dinner: Grilled shrimp with steamed green beans and couscous.
- Snack: Celery sticks with hummus.

Day 12

- Breakfast: Scrambled eggs with spinach and diced tomatoes.
- Lunch: Spinach and kale salad with grilled chicken, blueberries, and a lemon-tahini dressing.

- Dinner: Baked trout with a side of quinoa and roasted asparagus.
- Snack: Trail mix with cashews, raisins, and dark chocolate chips.

Day 13

- Breakfast: Whole-grain toast with mashed avocado and a poached egg.
- Lunch: Chickpea and quinoa salad with diced cucumber, red pepper, and a lemon-turmeric dressing.
- Dinner: Baked halibut with steamed broccoli and brown rice.
- Snack: Sliced cucumbers with tzatziki dip.

Day 14

- Breakfast: Chia seed pudding with sliced strawberries and a drizzle of honey.
- Lunch: Lentil and vegetable stir-fry with a sesame-ginger sauce served over brown rice.
- Dinner: Grilled chicken breast with roasted sweet potatoes and green beans.
- Snack: Mixed berries with a dollop of Greek yogurt.

CHAPTER THREE

Heavy metal detox breakfast recipes

1. Detox Green Smoothie

Start your day with a refreshing detox green smoothie packed with antioxidants and detoxifying ingredients.

Ingredients:

- 1 cup spinach leaves
- 1/2 cucumber, peeled and chopped
- 1/2 lemon, juiced
- 1/2 green apple, chopped
- 1/2 cup coconut water
- 1 tablespoon chia seeds
- Ice cubes (optional)

Instructions:

1. Place all ingredients in a blender.

2. Blend until smooth.

3. Add ice cubes for extra freshness.

4. Serve immediately.

Cooking Time: 5 minutes

2. Quinoa Breakfast Bowl

A protein-packed breakfast bowl loaded with quinoa and detoxifying fruits.

Ingredients:

- 1/2 cup cooked quinoa
- 1/2 cup mixed berries (blueberries, strawberries, raspberries)
- 1 tablespoon flaxseeds
- 1 tablespoon chopped almonds
- 1/2 teaspoon honey (optional)

Instructions:

1. In a bowl, layer cooked quinoa.

2. Top with mixed berries, flaxseeds, and chopped almonds.

3. Drizzle honey for sweetness if desired.

4. Mix and enjoy.

Cooking Time: 10 minutes (if quinoa is not pre-cooked)

3. Lemon-Ginger Detox Tea

A warm and soothing detox tea to kickstart your morning.

Ingredients:

- 1 cup hot water
- 1-inch piece of ginger, sliced
- 1/2 lemon, juiced
- 1 teaspoon honey (optional)

Instructions:

1. Pour hot water into a mug.

2. Add ginger slices and let steep for 3-5 minutes.

3. Stir in lemon juice and honey.

4. Sip slowly.

Cooking Time: 5 minutes

4. Chia Seed Pudding

A nutritious and fiber-rich pudding perfect for a heavy metal detox breakfast.

Ingredients:

- 2 tablespoons chia seeds
- 1/2 cup almond milk
- 1/2 teaspoon vanilla extract
- 1/4 cup mixed berries
- 1 teaspoon honey (optional)

Instructions:

1. Mix chia seeds, almond milk, and vanilla extract in a jar.

2. Refrigerate for at least 2 hours or overnight.

3. Top with mixed berries and honey.

4. Enjoy!

Cooking Time: 2 hours (overnight soak)

5. Detoxifying Oatmeal

A hearty and cleansing oatmeal recipe to fuel your day.

Ingredients:

- 1/2 cup rolled oats
- 1 cup water

- 1/2 teaspoon cinnamon
- 1/4 cup sliced banana
- 1 tablespoon chopped walnuts
- 1/2 teaspoon honey (optional)

Instructions:

1. Cook oats in water with cinnamon until creamy.

2. Top with sliced banana and chopped walnuts.

3. Drizzle honey for extra sweetness if desired.

4. Serve hot.

Cooking Time: 10 minutes

6. Berry Spinach Breakfast Salad

A unique and nutritious salad for those who prefer a savory breakfast.

Ingredients:

- 2 cups baby spinach leaves
- 1/2 cup mixed berries (blueberries, strawberries)
- 1/4 cup sliced almonds
- 1/4 cup feta cheese (optional)

- Balsamic vinaigrette dressing

Instructions:

1. Toss spinach, mixed berries, sliced almonds, and feta cheese (if using) in a bowl.

2. Drizzle with balsamic vinaigrette dressing.

3. Enjoy your breakfast salad!

Cooking Time: 10 minutes

7. Detoxifying Breakfast Burrito

A savory breakfast burrito filled with detoxifying ingredients.

Ingredients:

- 2 large eggs, scrambled
- 1/4 cup black beans, drained and rinsed
- 1/4 cup diced tomatoes
- 2 tablespoons chopped cilantro
- 1 whole-grain tortilla

Instructions:

1. Scramble the eggs until cooked.

2. Warm the tortilla.

3. Fill the tortilla with scrambled eggs, black beans, diced tomatoes, and cilantro.

4. Roll it up and enjoy.

Cooking Time: 15 minutes

8. Avocado and Salmon Toast

A delicious and omega-3 rich breakfast that supports heavy metal detox.

Ingredients:

- 1 slice whole-grain bread, toasted
- 1/2 avocado, mashed
- Smoked salmon slices
- Sliced cucumber
- Lemon zest

Instructions:

1. Spread mashed avocado on the toasted bread.

2. Top with smoked salmon, cucumber slices, and lemon zest.

3. Serve as an open-faced sandwich.

Cooking Time: 5 minutes

9. Detoxifying Greek Yogurt Parfait

A creamy and probiotic-rich breakfast parfait with detoxifying ingredients.

Ingredients:

- 1 cup Greek yogurt
- 1/4 cup mixed berries
- 1 tablespoon honey
- 1 tablespoon pumpkin seeds

Instructions:

1. Layer Greek yogurt in a glass or bowl.

2. Add mixed berries, drizzle with honey, and sprinkle with

pumpkin seeds.

3. Repeat layers as desired.

4. Enjoy your parfait!

Cooking Time: 5 minutes

10. Turmeric Scramble

A spicy and detoxifying twist on traditional scrambled eggs.

Ingredients:

- 2 large eggs, scrambled
- 1/4 teaspoon ground turmeric
- 1/4 teaspoon ground cumin
- A pinch of black pepper
- Chopped fresh cilantro
- Sliced avocado

Instructions:

1. Scramble the eggs with turmeric, cumin, and black pepper.

2. Cook until done.

3. Garnish with fresh cilantro and serve with sliced avocado.

Cooking Time: 10 minutes

Heavy Metal Detox Lunch Recipes

1. Detoxifying Lentil Soup

A hearty and flavorful soup loaded with fiber and detoxifying ingredients.

Ingredients:

- 1 cup green or brown lentils, rinsed
- 1 onion, chopped
- 2 carrots, diced
- 2 celery stalks, chopped
- 4 cups vegetable broth
- 1 teaspoon ground cumin
- 1/2 teaspoon turmeric
- Salt and pepper to taste
- Fresh parsley for garnish

Instructions:

1. In a large pot, sauté the onions, carrots, and celery until they soften.

2. Add lentils, vegetable broth, cumin, turmeric, salt, and pepper.

3. Simmer for 30-40 minutes until lentils are tender.

4. Garnish with fresh parsley and serve hot.

Cooking Time: 45 minutes

2. Spinach and Chickpea Salad

A protein-packed salad with spinach and chickpeas to support your detox efforts.

Ingredients:

- 2 cups baby spinach leaves
- 1 cup cooked chickpeas
- 1/2 red bell pepper, diced
- 1/4 red onion, thinly sliced
- 1/4 cup crumbled feta cheese (optional)
- Balsamic vinaigrette dressing

Instructions:

1. Toss spinach, chickpeas, red bell pepper, and red onion in a bowl.

2. Top with crumbled feta cheese (if using).

3. Drizzle with balsamic vinaigrette dressing.

4. Enjoy your protein-packed salad.

Cooking Time: 10 minutes (if chickpeas are pre-cooked)

3. Detoxifying Cauliflower Rice Bowl

A low-carb and nutrient-rich lunch option packed with detoxifying ingredients.

Ingredients:

- 2 cups cauliflower rice
- 1 cup steamed broccoli florets
- 1/2 cup diced cucumber
- 1/2 cup shredded carrots
- 1/4 cup sliced almonds
- 2 tablespoons tahini dressing

Instructions:

1. Sauté cauliflower rice until tender.

2. Arrange cauliflower rice in a bowl.

3. Top with steamed broccoli, diced cucumber, shredded carrots, and sliced almonds.

4. Drizzle with tahini dressing.

5. Enjoy your cauliflower rice bowl.

Cooking Time: 15 minutes (if cauliflower rice is not premade)

4. Detoxifying Quinoa Salad

A versatile and nutrient-packed salad that promotes detoxification.

Ingredients:

- 1 cup cooked quinoa
- 1/2 cup diced cucumber
- 1/2 cup cherry tomatoes, halved
- 1/4 cup chopped fresh mint
- 1/4 cup crumbled goat cheese (optional)
- Lemon-turmeric dressing

Instructions:

1. In a bowl, combine cooked quinoa, diced cucumber, cherry tomatoes, and chopped fresh mint.

2. Top with crumbled goat cheese (if using).

3. Drizzle with lemon-turmeric dressing.

4. Toss well and serve.

Cooking Time: 15 minutes (if quinoa is not pre-cooked)

5. Detoxifying Sushi Bowl

A deconstructed sushi bowl with detoxifying ingredients for a satisfying lunch.

Ingredients:

- 1 cup cooked brown rice
- 4-6 sushi-grade nori seaweed sheets, torn into small pieces
- 1/2 cucumber, diced
- 1/2 avocado, sliced
- 4-6 cooked shrimp or crab sticks
- Pickled ginger and low-sodium soy sauce for serving

Instructions:

1. In a bowl, layer cooked brown rice.

2. Top with torn nori seaweed sheets, diced cucumber, avocado slices, and cooked shrimp or crab sticks.

3. Serve with pickled ginger and low-sodium soy sauce.

Cooking Time: 15 minutes (if rice is not pre-cooked)

6. Detoxifying Turmeric Lentil Salad

A colorful and anti-inflammatory salad packed with detoxifying ingredients.

Ingredients:

- 1 cup cooked red lentils
- 1/2 cup diced bell peppers (a mix of colors)
- 1/2 cup grated carrots
- 1/4 cup chopped fresh cilantro
- Turmeric-tahini dressing

Instructions:

1. In a bowl, combine cooked red lentils, diced bell peppers, grated carrots, and chopped fresh cilantro.

2. Drizzle with turmeric-tahini dressing.

3. Toss well and serve.

Cooking Time: 20 minutes (if lentils are not pre-cooked)

7. Detoxifying Cabbage and Avocado Slaw

A crunchy and creamy slaw loaded with detoxifying ingredients.

Ingredients:

- 2 cups shredded green cabbage
- 1/2 avocado, mashed
- 1/4 cup diced red onion
- 1/4 cup chopped fresh parsley
- Lemon-garlic dressing

Instructions:

1. In a bowl, combine shredded green cabbage, mashed avocado, diced red onion, and chopped fresh parsley.

2. Drizzle with lemon-garlic dressing.

3. Toss well and serve.

Cooking Time: 10 minutes

8. Detoxifying Sweet Potato and Kale Salad

A nutrient-rich salad featuring sweet potatoes and kale, perfect for supporting heavy metal detox.

Ingredients:

- 2 cups chopped kale leaves
- 1 roasted sweet potato, diced
- 1/4 cup pomegranate seeds
- 1/4 cup chopped walnuts
- Balsamic vinaigrette dressing

Instructions:

1. Massage kale leaves with a bit of dressing to soften.

2. In a bowl, combine chopped kale, diced roasted sweet potato, pomegranate seeds, and chopped walnuts.

3. Drizzle with balsamic vinaigrette dressing.

4. Toss well and serve.

Cooking Time: 30 minutes (if sweet potato is not pre-roasted)

9. Detoxifying Chickpea and Veggie Wrap

A portable and satisfying wrap filled with detoxifying ingredients.

Ingredients:

- 1 whole-grain tortilla
- 1/2 cup hummus
- 1/2 cup diced cucumber
- 1/2 cup diced bell peppers (a mix of colors)
- 1/4 cup shredded carrots
- Fresh cilantro leaves

Instructions:

1. Spread hummus evenly on the whole-grain tortilla.

2. Layer with diced cucumber, diced bell peppers, shredded carrots, and fresh cilantro leaves.

3. Roll up the tortilla and cut it in half.

4. Enjoy your detoxifying wrap.

Cooking Time: 10 minutes

10. Detoxifying Lemon-Garlic Salmon

A flavorful and protein-rich salmon dish with detoxifying lemon and garlic.

Ingredients:

- 1 salmon fillet
- Juice of 1 lemon
- 2 garlic cloves, minced
- 1 teaspoon olive oil
- Salt and pepper to taste
- Steamed broccoli and quinoa for serving

Instructions:

1. Preheat your oven to 375°F (190°C).

2. Place the salmon fillet on a baking sheet.

3. Mix lemon juice, minced garlic, olive oil, salt, and pepper in a bowl.

4. Pour the lemon-garlic mixture over the salmon.

5. Bake for 15-20 minutes until the salmon is cooked through.

6. Serve with steamed broccoli and quinoa.

Cooking Time: 20-25 minutes

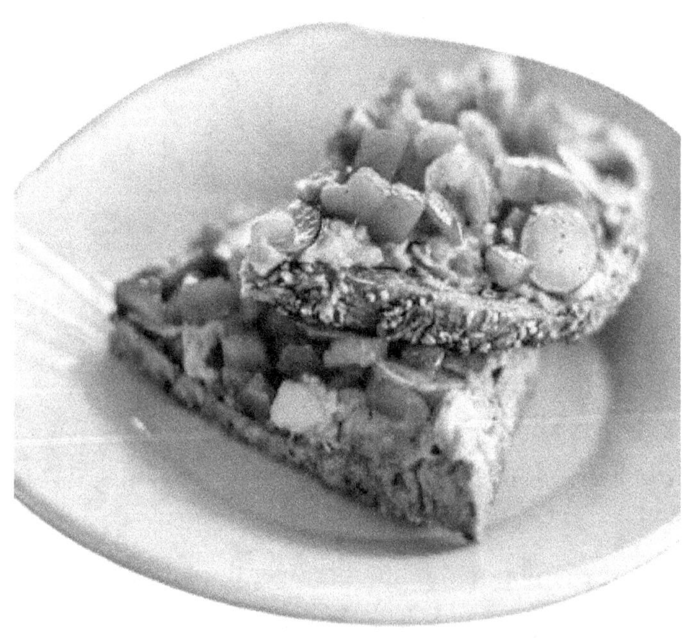

CHAPTER FOUR

Heavy Metal Detox Dinner Recipes

1. Detoxifying Miso Soup

A warm and soothing miso soup with seaweed and tofu for a detoxifying dinner.

Ingredients:

- 4 cups vegetable broth
- 2 tablespoons miso paste
- 1 sheet nori seaweed, torn into small pieces
- 1 cup diced tofu
- 1 cup sliced mushrooms
- 2 green onions, thinly sliced

Instructions:

1. In a pot, heat vegetable broth over medium heat.

2. Dissolve miso paste in a small amount of hot broth and then add it to the pot.

3. Add torn nori seaweed, diced tofu, sliced mushrooms, and green onions.

4. Simmer for 10-15 minutes.

5. Serve hot.

Cooking Time: 20 minutes

2. Detoxifying Turmeric and Ginger Rice Bowl

A flavorful and anti-inflammatory rice bowl with turmeric and ginger.

Ingredients:

- 1 cup cooked brown rice
- 1 cup steamed broccoli
- 1/2 cup diced bell peppers (a mix of colors)
- 1/2 cup sliced snap peas
- 1 tablespoon chopped fresh cilantro
- Turmeric-ginger dressing

Instructions:

1. In a bowl, layer cooked brown rice.

2. Top with steamed broccoli, diced bell peppers, sliced snap peas, and chopped cilantro.

3. Drizzle with turmeric-ginger dressing.

4. Toss well and serve.

Cooking Time: 15 minutes (if rice is not pre-cooked)

3. Detoxifying Chickpea and Spinach Curry

A fragrant and comforting curry with chickpeas and spinach, rich in detoxifying spices.

Ingredients:

-   1 cup cooked chickpeas
-   2 cups fresh spinach leaves
-   1 onion, finely chopped
-   2 cloves garlic, minced
-   1-inch piece of ginger, grated
-   1 can (14 oz) diced tomatoes
-   1 tablespoon curry powder
-   1/2 teaspoon ground turmeric
-   Salt and pepper to taste
-   2 tablespoons coconut oil

Instructions:

1. In a large skillet, heat coconut oil over medium heat.

2. Add chopped onion, minced garlic, and grated ginger.

Sauté until fragrant.

3. Stir in curry powder and ground turmeric.

4. Add diced tomatoes and cook for 5 minutes.

5. Add cooked chickpeas and fresh spinach. Cook until spinach wilts.

6. Season with salt and pepper.

7. Serve hot with brown rice or quinoa.

Cooking Time: 30 minutes (if chickpeas are not pre-cooked)

4. Detoxifying Lemon-Herb Baked Cod

A light and flavorful baked cod dish with detoxifying lemon and herbs.

Ingredients:

- 2 cod fillets
- Juice of 1 lemon
- 2 cloves garlic, minced
- 1 teaspoon fresh thyme leaves
- 1 teaspoon fresh rosemary leaves

- Salt and pepper to taste

- Olive oil for drizzling

Instructions:

1. Preheat your oven to 375°F (190°C).

2. Place cod fillets on a baking sheet.

3. Drizzle with olive oil and sprinkle with minced garlic, thyme, rosemary, salt, and pepper.

4. Squeeze lemon juice over the top.

5. Bake for 15-20 minutes until the cod is cooked through.

6. Serve hot with steamed asparagus or a side salad.

Cooking Time: 20-25 minutes

5. Detoxifying Quinoa and Vegetable Stir-Fry

A colorful and nutrient-packed vegetable stir-fry with quinoa.

Ingredients:

- 1 cup cooked quinoa

- 1 cup mixed vegetables (broccoli, bell peppers, snap

peas)

- 1/2 cup sliced mushrooms

- 2 cloves garlic, minced

- 1 tablespoon low-sodium soy sauce or tamari

- 1/2 teaspoon ground ginger

- 1 tablespoon sesame oil

Instructions:

1. Heat sesame oil in a large skillet over medium-high heat.

2. Add minced garlic and sliced mushrooms. Sauté until mushrooms start to brown.

3. Add mixed vegetables and stir-fry until tender.

4. Stir in cooked quinoa, low-sodium soy sauce or tamari, and ground ginger.

5. Cook for an additional 2-3 minutes.

6. Serve hot.

Cooking Time: 20 minutes (if quinoa is not pre-cooked)

6. Detoxifying Sweet Potato and Black Bean Chili

A hearty and fiber-rich chili featuring sweet potatoes and black beans.

Ingredients:

- 2 sweet potatoes, diced
- 1 can (15 oz) black beans, drained and rinsed
- 1 can (14 oz) diced tomatoes
- 1 onion, chopped
- 2 cloves garlic, minced
- 1 tablespoon chili powder
- 1 teaspoon ground cumin
- Salt and pepper to taste
- Chopped fresh cilantro for garnish

Instructions:

1. In a large pot, sauté chopped onion and minced garlic until translucent.

2. Add diced sweet potatoes, black beans, diced tomatoes, chili powder, ground cumin, salt, and pepper.

3. Simmer for 20-25 minutes until sweet potatoes are tender.

4. Garnish with chopped fresh cilantro.

5. Serve hot.

Cooking Time: 30 minutes

7. Detoxifying Lemon-Dill Grilled Salmon

A flavorful and omega-3 rich grilled salmon dish with lemon and dill.

Ingredients:

- 2 salmon fillets
- Juice of 1 lemon
- 2 tablespoons fresh dill, chopped
- 2 cloves garlic, minced
- Salt and pepper to taste
- Olive oil for grilling

Instructions:

1. Preheat your grill to medium-high heat.

2. Season salmon fillets with minced garlic, chopped dill, salt, pepper, and lemon juice.

3. Drizzle with olive oil.

4. Grill for 5-6 minutes per side until salmon is cooked through.

5. Serve hot with steamed green beans or a side salad.

Cooking Time: 15-20 minutes

8. Detoxifying Turmeric and Coconut Lentil Curry

A creamy and anti-inflammatory lentil curry with turmeric and coconut milk.

Ingredients:

- 1 cup red lentils
- 1 can (14 oz) coconut milk
- 1 onion, finely chopped
- 2 cloves garlic, minced
- 1-inch piece of ginger, grated
- 1 tablespoon curry powder
- 1/2 teaspoon ground turmeric
- Salt and pepper to taste
- Fresh cilantro leaves for garnish

Instructions:

1. In a large pot, sauté chopped onion, minced garlic, and grated ginger until fragrant.

2. Stir in curry powder and ground turmeric.

3. Add red lentils and coconut milk.

4. Simmer for 20-25 minutes until lentils are soft.

5. Season with salt and pepper.

6. Garnish with fresh cilantro leaves.

7. Serve hot with brown rice or quinoa.

Cooking Time: 30 minutes

9. Detoxifying Cucumber and Avocado Gazpacho

Ingredients:

- 2 cucumbers, peeled and chopped
- 1 avocado, peeled and diced
- 1/2 cup fresh cilantro leaves
- 2 cloves garlic, minced

- Juice of 2 limes
- 1/4 cup low-fat Greek yogurt (optional)
- Salt and pepper to taste
- Crushed red pepper flakes for garnish

Instructions:

1. In a blender, combine chopped cucumbers, diced avocado, fresh cilantro leaves, minced garlic, lime juice, and Greek yogurt (if using).

2. Blend until smooth.

3. Season with salt and pepper.

4. Chill in the refrigerator for at least 1 hour before serving.

5. Garnish with crushed red pepper flakes.

6. Serve chilled.

Cooking Time: 10 minutes

10. Detoxifying Stuffed Bell Peppers

A nutritious and colorful dinner option with detoxifying ingredients.

Ingredients:

- 4 bell peppers (red, yellow, or green)
- 1 cup quinoa, cooked
- 1 can (15 oz) black beans, drained and rinsed
- 1 cup corn kernels
- 1 cup diced tomatoes
- 1/2 cup diced red onion
- 1/2 teaspoon ground cumin
- 1/2 teaspoon chili powder
- Salt and pepper to taste
- Shredded cheddar cheese (optional)

Instructions:

1. Preheat your oven to 375°F (190°C).

2. Cut the tops off the bell peppers and remove the seeds.

3. In a bowl, combine cooked quinoa, black beans, corn kernels, diced tomatoes, diced red onion, ground cumin,

chili powder, salt, and pepper.

4. Stuff each bell pepper with the quinoa mixture.

5. Place stuffed peppers in a baking dish.

6. Bake for 30-35 minutes until peppers are tender.

7. If desired, sprinkle shredded cheddar cheese on top and bake for an additional 5 minutes until melted.

8. Serve hot.

Cooking Time: 40-45 minutes

Heavy Metal Detox Snacks Recipes

1. Detoxifying Green Smoothie Bowl

A refreshing and nutritious smoothie bowl filled with detoxifying ingredients for a satisfying snack.

Ingredients:

- 1 cup spinach leaves
- 1/2 banana
- 1/2 cup almond milk
- 1 tablespoon chia seeds
- Sliced kiwi, berries, and granola for topping

Instructions:

1. Blend spinach, banana, and almond milk until smooth.

2. Pour into a bowl.

3. Top with chia seeds, sliced kiwi, berries, and granola.

4. Enjoy your green smoothie bowl.

Cooking Time: 5 minutes

2. Detoxifying Cucumber and Hummus Bites

A simple and crunchy snack that pairs detoxifying cucumbers with creamy hummus.

Ingredients:

- 1 cucumber, sliced into rounds
- 1/4 cup hummus
- Fresh dill or parsley for garnish

Instructions:

1. Arrange cucumber slices on a plate.

2. Place a dollop of hummus on each cucumber round.

3. Garnish with fresh dill or parsley.

4. Serve chilled.

Cooking Time: 5 minutes

3. Detoxifying Chia Seed Pudding

A fiber-rich pudding made with chia seeds and detoxifying fruits for a satisfying snack.

Ingredients:

- 2 tablespoons chia seeds
- 1/2 cup almond milk
- 1/4 cup mixed berries
- 1/4 teaspoon vanilla extract
- Drizzle of honey (optional)

Instructions:

1. Mix chia seeds, almond milk, vanilla extract, and a drizzle of honey (if desired) in a jar.

2. Refrigerate for at least 2 hours or overnight.

3. Top with mixed berries before serving.

4. Enjoy your chia seed pudding.

Cooking Time: 2 hours (overnight soak)

4. Detoxifying Beet and Carrot Chips

Homemade vegetable chips made from detoxifying beets and carrots.

Ingredients:

-   2 beets, thinly sliced
-   2 carrots, thinly sliced
-   Olive oil
-   Sea salt
-   Ground black pepper
-   Dried rosemary (optional)

Instructions:

1. Preheat your oven to 325°F (160°C).

2. Toss beet and carrot slices with olive oil, sea salt, ground black pepper, and dried rosemary (if using).

3. Spread the slices on a baking sheet.

4. Bake for 20-25 minutes until crisp.

5. Let cool before serving.

Cooking Time: 25 minutes

5. Detoxifying Greek Yogurt Parfait

A creamy and probiotic-rich parfait with detoxifying ingredients.

Ingredients:

- 1 cup Greek yogurt
- 1/4 cup mixed berries
- 1 tablespoon honey
- 1 tablespoon chopped walnuts

Instructions:

1. Layer Greek yogurt in a glass or bowl.

2. Add mixed berries, drizzle with honey, and sprinkle with chopped walnuts.

3. Repeat layers as desired.

4. Enjoy your Greek yogurt parfait.

Cooking Time: 5 minutes

6. Detoxifying Almond and Turmeric Roasted Chickpeas

A crunchy and protein-packed snack with detoxifying turmeric and almonds.

Ingredients:

- 1 can (15 oz) chickpeas, drained and rinsed
- 1 tablespoon olive oil
- 1 teaspoon ground turmeric
- 1/4 cup chopped almonds
- Sea salt to taste

Instructions:

1. Preheat your oven to 400°F (200°C).

2. Pat chickpeas dry with a paper towel.

3. Toss chickpeas with olive oil, ground turmeric, chopped almonds, and sea salt.

4. Spread the chickpeas on a baking sheet.

5. Roast for 25-30 minutes until crispy.

6. Let cool before snacking.

Cooking Time: 30 minutes

7. Detoxifying Mixed Nut Trail Mix

A nutrient-packed trail mix loaded with detoxifying nuts and dried fruits.

Ingredients:

- 1/2 cup almonds
- 1/2 cup walnuts
- 1/4 cup dried cranberries
- 1/4 cup dried apricots, chopped
- 1/4 cup pumpkin seeds
- 1/4 cup dark chocolate chips (optional)

Instructions:

1. Mix almonds, walnuts, dried cranberries, dried apricots, pumpkin seeds, and dark chocolate chips (if using) in a bowl.

2. Store in an airtight container for a convenient snack.

Cooking Time: 5 minutes

8. Detoxifying Sliced Apple and Peanut Butter

A classic and satisfying snack pairing crisp apple slices with creamy peanut butter.

Ingredients:

- 1 apple, sliced
- 2 tablespoons peanut butter

Instructions:

1. Slice the apple into wedges.

2. Dip apple slices into peanut butter.

3. Enjoy your apple and peanut butter snack.

Cooking Time: 5 minutes

9. Detoxifying Roasted Edamame

A protein-packed snack with roasted edamame and detoxifying spices.

Ingredients:

- 1 cup frozen edamame, thawed
- 1 teaspoon olive oil

- 1/2 teaspoon ground cumin

- 1/2 teaspoon chili powder

- Salt and pepper to taste

Instructions:

1. Preheat your oven to 375°F (190°C).

2. Toss thawed edamame with olive oil, ground cumin, chili powder, salt, and pepper.

3. Spread on a baking sheet.

4. Roast for 15-20 minutes until crispy.

5. Let cool before snacking.

Cooking Time: 20 minutes

10. Detoxifying Chocolate Avocado Mousse

A creamy and guilt-free chocolate mousse made with detoxifying avocados.

Ingredients:

- 2 ripe avocados

- 1/4 cup cocoa powder

-   1/4 cup honey or maple syrup

-   1 teaspoon vanilla extract

-   A pinch of sea salt

-   Fresh berries for garnish

Instructions:

1. Blend avocados, cocoa powder, honey or maple syrup, vanilla extract, and a pinch of sea salt until smooth.

2. Chill in the refrigerator for at least 1 hour.

3. Garnish with fresh berries before serving.

4. Enjoy your chocolate avocado mousse.

Cooking Time: 5 minutes (plus chilling time)

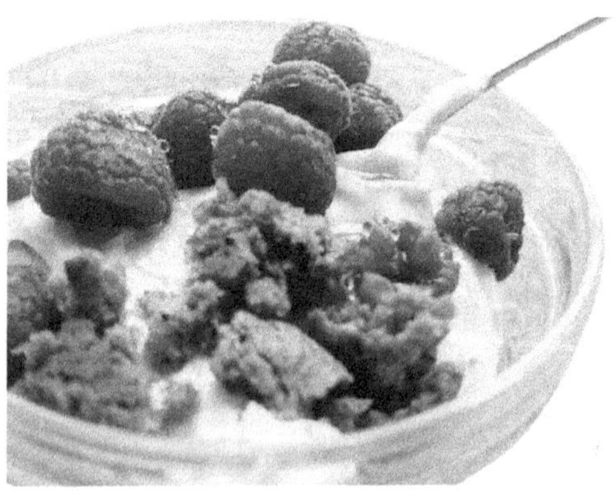

CONCLUSION

In conclusion, the heavy metal detox diet is a holistic approach to wellness that emphasizes the removal of harmful heavy metals from the body while promoting overall health and well-being. This dietary regimen focuses on incorporating foods rich in antioxidants, vitamins, and minerals that support the body's natural detoxification processes.

Through careful meal planning and the inclusion of specific detoxifying ingredients, people can minimize their exposure to heavy metals and help the body eliminate any accumulated toxins.

The benefits of a heavy metal detox diet are multifaceted. First and foremost, it can aid in reducing the risk of heavy metal toxicity, which can lead to a range of health issues, including neurological problems, organ damage, and chronic diseases.

By adopting this diet, individuals can take proactive steps to safeguard their health and protect themselves from the harmful effects of heavy metals.

Additionally, a heavy metal detox diet can contribute to overall wellness. The emphasis on whole foods, fresh fruits and vegetables, and nutrient-dense ingredients provides the body with essential vitamins and minerals. This can boost the immune system, increase energy levels, and improve overall vitality.

Moreover, the heavy metal detox diet encourages mindfulness about food choices and sources. It prompts individuals to be conscious of where their food comes from, emphasizing organic and sustainably sourced ingredients. This not only supports personal health but also promotes environmentally responsible practices.

Incorporating heavy metal detox principles into one's dietary routine can be a gradual process, and it may require consultation with a healthcare professional or nutritionist for personalized guidance. However, the potential benefits are well worth the effort, as they encompass not only detoxification but also long-term health and vitality.

By combining these elements, individuals can optimize their health and reduce the risk of heavy metal exposure, ultimately leading to a happier and healthier life.